How I Lost 70 Pounds Without Exercise...And Lived To Tell About It

by Mark Druckmiller

<u>Acknowledgments</u>

Thanks to my family, Jd, Alexa, Adam, and Connie for putting up with my strange cooking, loading up the kitchen with strange foods and boxes, and generally putting up with me all these years.

Thanks to my Facebook friends and my friends in real life for all the encouragement and support, mostly during the bad days where my weight would fluctuate.

Thanks to the weight loss professionals that I've dealt with over the years and the ones that I'm using now, Mary, Kim, Mickey, Vicki, and Pam.

...and thanks to Irving T Duck.

Table of Contents

Why SHOULD you read this book? How to tick off lawyers.

The past - what did/didn't/sorta worked

What Is Different Now and How I Started

Mark's Basic Idea Number One: Either go to a clinic, company, community group, hospital, or join a group of friends or co-workers in a weight-loss plan together.

Mark's Basic Idea Number Two: Bring attention to yourself and declare yourself as being on a weight-loss program using social media.

Mark's Basic Idea Number Three: Set a goal AND a reward for losing weight.

As part of the goal, set up a big REWARD or BET that if you complete the goal, you will buy something nice, or do something that you've always wanted to do, or something else.

Mark's Basic Idea Number Four: Track what you eat, when, and how much, and track what you weigh.

Some of the science, good, bad, and otherwise

Mark's Basic Idea Number Five: Eat too much or without limits and you'll gain weight.

Mark's Basic Idea Number Six: Almost anything sweet is NOT your friend.

Mark's Basic Idea Number Seven: Carbs are not your friend.

Mark's Basic Idea Number Eight: Most vegetables are okay, the more the better.

Mark's Basic Idea Number Nine: Fat doesn't necessarily go directly into your own fat, but go ahead and load up on protein

Mark's Basic Idea Number Ten: Stay off salt/sodium

Mark's Basic Idea Number Eleven: Exercise is good for you of course, but it's not the total solution

Mark's Basic Idea Number Twelve: To maintain your sanity, one "cheat meal" a week can help make the long-running process of weight loss easier to continue

Mark's Basic Idea Number Thirteen: Get a good scale, but only weigh yourself every few days or every WEEK, don't weigh yourself every day

What to do now that you're there?

Epilogue:

References, resources, and places where I found stuff about diets and dieting:

Why SHOULD you read this book? How to tick off lawyers.

First things first. I am NOT a doctor. I am NOT a nutritionist. I am not a body builder. I am not a diet counselor. I am not an exercise guru. I am not a health nut.

I'm saying this as to not be glib and throwing disclaimers out there to keep the lawyers away, but here's the real truth. I'm a guy who actually lost 70 pounds. I lived through it. I got to see what works and what doesn't.

I'm actually trying to lose MORE weight, but I thought I'd share some information, maybe avoid some of the big mistakes on how to lose weight and what happens if you do or DON'T do these things.

What am I? I'm a real estate agent. Actually, I've been in real estate for five years and in information technology for over 30 years. Yup, a computer geek. I have had no nutritional training beyond what most of the public does, reading books and hitting websites. I've never even taken a biology class in school   What do I have for training on diet and foods and exercise? NONE. But I feel qualified just to tell you what I did and how it worked for me.

That's all.

So it's not a "how to lose weight" book, but a "here's what happened to me when I tried to lose weight" book. Big difference.

You may get ideas. You might get inspired. You may want to change your mind about your body habits and do something right for a change. You may at least avoid doing some bad things (like eating bad foods) and that may make you better in the long run. You might seek professional help. You may do nothing.

Here's a list of disclaimers for now and being brutally honest.

- You may lose weight easily.
- You may lose weight with great difficulty, intense depression, and it may take forever.

- You may feel great.
- You may feel like you got smacked by a cement truck.
- You may feel refreshed and have more energy.
- You may feel like you've been run through a wood chipper.
- You may live forever.
- You may die a quick and painful death, pass out frequently, go into cardiac arrest, or be committed to a mental institution.
- You may feel more emotionally enthusiastic, make new friends, and be the life of the party.
- You may collapse in a heap on your couch and feel like crap.
- Your guts may explode, you may break out in spots, and you might hear colors.
- Doctors are going to look at this book, and many of them may say it violates everything about nutrition, general health, and science for that matter.

There are no guarantees, no promises, much of my information is purely anecdotal, but I will supply some links to the sources I used for credible and verifiable information. The more you can check and verify and corroborate the better.

Now while I stated earlier that I'm still losing weight, I've also read up and plan to implement things that I've seen work for others in order to keep weight off after you lose it.

The reason I put this out, not being a credentialed, degreed, or certified expert is mostly because many of these experts have not actually lived through BEING obese, overweight, or close to death. Many have good ideas, or have lots of good information, and have track records of helping people. But I would tend to feel more confident and trusting of someone that actually endured and underwent the process of actually losing weight and all the difficulties one can go through.

But I wanted to present a view of what it was like as the one DOING the weight loss. I get to explain what was going on in my head, my justifications, my reasons, my emotions, my successes and my FAILURES.

That's also the reason this book is moderately priced. That is, you might need to spend more time, effort, and even money to get into some of these things I've used to lose weight. It's just advice or at least just a good start.

About the "without exercise" part: What that means is that I didn't start any new exercise regime, or take up walking, jogging, or some other organized exercise on top of my basic physical activity. I'm a part-time musician and I carry a lot of gear weekly when practicing or playing gigs. But I didn't start anything new. More on that later.

Ultimately it is this: I WILL NOT SWEAR THIS WILL WORK FOR EVERYONE. SOME of these things worked for ME.

The past - what did/didn't/sorta worked

Just a smattering of incidents and observations through my life.

1970's - I was pretty overweight as a kid and a teen. My brothers weren't, which I couldn't figure out. I endured some pretty merciless teasing from my older brother, but kids tease each other all the time. Probably the most I weighed was around 220 as a 6 foot tall late teen with a 38-inch waist. I was pretty averse to sports, even though I played 4-H softball (not that strenuous) but I was invited to try out for track and cross-country. In grade school, I participated, but could not make it around the 440-yard long run around the football field. In cross country, on a 4-mile run, I barely made it to one mile, and walked the entire remainder of the trip. Very bad. To this day, and with such bad memories, I'm pretty much exercise-averse, or that is, I hate any aerobic activity. I never liked the huffing and puffing, breathing heavily, and never liked all the pain and being uncomfortable and all the sweating. Hate sweating.

1980's - Amazingly, I think I did a 180-degree turnaround for the early part of the decade while I was a college student at the University of Illinois in Champaign and Urbana. Notice that. Champaign AND Urbana. My classes were mostly at the northeast end of the campus (Urbana) , but my dormitory was at the SOUTHWEST end of the campus (Champaign). Being a typical college student, I'd get up, skip breakfast, do a fast walk to my classes, and my meals usually consisted of a lunch salad and a bagel, evening meals were mostly that as well. I think it was mostly that I could usually get through the salad bar faster than the "hot meal" line. Whatever happened there did something to me, I lost about 50 pounds (weighed about 170), and stayed there for a few years.

After getting married in 1986, I think I hovered around 190 to 210 up until my first child was born in 1998.

Life got changed quick. As our lives got busier, my body chemistry and metabolism changed as things do when you get older. However, I always snored and in 2000 was officially diagnosed as having sleep apnea. Being around 240 pounds didn't help either. I did a lot of the home cooking, so to

speak, in which I would cook stuff that my kids love, like noodles and other pasta. I had the sleep apnea surgery, basically fixing my deviated septum and getting a UPPP (Uvulopalatopharyngoplasty)
or that is, getting my little hangy thing in the back of my mouth removed as well as widening that area back there.   My snoring stopped, but did it really help anything else? I still weighed around 240.

In 2001, we moved from suburban Atlanta to suburban Chicago. During our first winter there, I lost about 20 pounds from a combination of working weird schedules at home, driving to and from daycare for the kids, and shoveling out a ton of snow (it WAS a bad winter, snow-wise). I fell to 220 pounds.

In 2002, we moved again, and this time around, I dealt with two small children, my wife with a stressful job, and dealing with a very crooked "house builder" (I used that in quotes as this is how bad the situation was, he wasn't licensed and spent more time in court than building houses). My stress level increased, I was cooking and eating food for comfort.

As of 2004 I weighed 275 pounds.

My sleep apnea had come back with a vengeance, I was tired a lot, falling asleep at my desk, immediately crashing in my Lay-Z-Boy recliner after putting the kids to bed at 8PM, or even earlier. I was a lot more tired, I was seeking other things to compensate for that. I had found the Atkins low-carb diet and decided to give that a try. That actually did work for awhile.

I got down to 240 pounds in early 2005, but stopped the Atkins diet when I had a medical incident and was hospitalized. I was also put on two blood pressure medicines.

I had gotten up to 290 pounds by 2010, managed to lose about 20 pounds and was down to one blood pressure medication. During that time I saw two "nutritionists". I put that in quotes as well mostly because my "seeing" them consisted of MONTHLY appointments. I'd get a stack of handouts about proper nutrition or short bits of advice, but no real ACTIVE engagement, or just telling me "eat about 1800 calories a day instead of 2400". But that was it.

Then I got the wake-up calls, or as I call it "the come to Jesus" moments.

In late October of 2012, my sleep apnea was worse. I was having a hard time keeping awake while ON THE ROAD. A couple more incidents up through 2014 was scary enough.

I was trying to cut down in other ways, but not totally committed. For lunch I'd have pre-packaged frozen meals (Weight Watchers, Lean Cuisine, even Atkins had a line of meals). I had signed up and used Weight Watchers online "point" system to try and do a program on my own. That didn't really help.

Then the big thing hit.

A blood test was showing I had encountered liver damage. I was at 322 pounds. I was having real problems staying awake at times where I needed to be awake. I was wearing 44-inch waist pants...and they were tight. I play in two classic rock bands and just transporting my own instruments wore me out just BEFORE even playing. I really had problems trying to help load up the rest of the band gear.

That was it. I had to do something different.

So at least I didn't have a heart attack, or stroke, or choked on a sandwich. Nothing like that, but knowing you're actually getting REAL testable and verifiable organ damage was enough to convince me something had to change.

What Is Different Now and How I Started

I'm going to go over a few of important things about what is different now about my weight loss routine compared to previous years.

If you drop the book after these few points, that's okay, I've done my job. I hate diet books that ramble on for hundreds of pages, either going heavy into the science, or keep repeating some of the same stuff over and over and don't encapsulate the needed information into a simple nugget.

I kept on seeing a particular "weight loss clinic" advertise a lot on local TV. I went in and started in on their program.

Now before we go any further, this isn't necessarily me telling you, "just go to a weight loss clinic". It's a lot more because part of what I can tell you is different about doing this then about going on your own is the first of my basic ideas.

Mark's Basic Idea Number One: Either go to a clinic, company, community group, hospital, or join a group of friends or co-workers in a weight-loss plan together.

The basic reason I suggest this will help and is different than doing other things is that you will have someone help monitor, support, offer advice, or even brainstorm with you on things you can or should to do to lose weight. That is, "going alone" had some short mild successes, but was lacking in encouragement, or information, or tracking progress and lead to MAJOR FAILURE.

I went to a clinic that has been in operation for over 20 years with proven success (it's only in my part of the country, and for now while I'm still on their program, I do not wish to share the name of it for now, and of course, I hate lawyers). That helped me because I went in 3 times a week to check progress, get information on what I should eat and shouldn't eat, and they tracked weight, measurements, and blood pressure. (And of course I had to pee on a stick to keep me in check and not burn muscle tissue instead of fat...)

That's working for me.

As for you, you can do the same, but you can also try Weight Watchers, but actually GO to their offices, go to meetings, and get them to actively weigh you and get their advice and support on weight loss. I tried the "Online Weight Watchers" program where I would try and follow their system where you logged "points" for what you ate. If you ate something not considered healthy (a piece of cake) that would be more points than if you ate something healthy (like a bunch of carrots). You could eat only up to a certain amount of points per day, and that total amount was based on what their website calculated was a good "limit" for you. The problems with that program was that the points they had calculated for me actually was too much, or that is I had no problems staying under the limit, but it didn't really make a dent. Their website was great, it could actually calculate a lot of the different foods for you and give you a reasonable figure for their "point" system, but I think the only way it would have worked for me is if I took their daily limit number and eat to a lower total per day. So with little to no results, I didn't feel I was getting anything out of it, including any encouragement. I feel that if I attended an actual Weight Watchers facility and went to their meetings, I'd have much better luck.

Jenny Craig is similar, they have both in-person clinics and do-it-yourself programs, but again I suggest the latter, as I strongly urge you get support.

Those aren't the only ones, either, you can also look at your local hospitals and recreation centers and they may offer similar programs where you can meet fairly frequently. Daily might be too often, a few times weekly would be great, weekly would barely be enough, anything longer than that is way too long.

You can even check to see if a group of employees would be interested in trying to lose weight together, either getting together to figure out a "proper diet" (more on that later) or choosing to follow some established ones such as the Weight Watchers online or similar, but adapting it to use together.

The clinics and classes help with the info, but any group will help you with monitoring and tracking. Most of all, you will NEED support. I mean it.

I'm a bit of a shy guy at work and keep to myself, mostly because many of my casual interests and hobbies are nothing like that of my co-workers. But in the different employers I've worked at, many did have formal or informal weight-loss groups.

In my case, the clinic did the following things for me:
1) Set up a program of what I can eat and not eat, when, how often, and other guidelines.
2) I had to write down what I ate every meal, every day.
3) I had to come in 3 times a week (the clinic was open from Monday through Saturday) to get weighed, they took a look at what I ate since the last visit, and took my blood pressure.
4) They offer advice and help on questions on what works and what doesn't, or give you a stern warning if you're wandering off eating bad stuff...

So if we translate this into something we can all implement if you do this as your own group (co-workers, friends), it's

1) Adopt a program of specific eating or dieting that has had proven results.
2) Write down what you eat and share with the group.
3) Meet together to discuss, cheer, or commiserate on everyone's progress.
4) Discuss new goals for the next meeting or next week, or whatever, including other strategies to try in your weight loss program.

What else seems to work? As much as I've mentioned doing this as a group, this is something you can either use in place of or ADD to the above working with a clinic or group:

Mark's Basic Idea Number Two: Bring attention to yourself and declare yourself as being on a weight-loss program using social media.

That is, if you like being an attention whore on Facebook, go for it! I'm not just posting updates to my personal timeline, I've actually created a separate fan page called "Watch Mark Lose 100 Pounds" (https://www.facebook.com/MarkLoses100lbs). I've probably not posted as much as I really want to, just being a busy guy, I post some comments on how I'm doing, but I mostly post a graph roughly once a week to show how I'm doing.   What does this do? Your friends and relatives, like those that are far away, will encourage you and give you some support. The nice compliments aren't bad either. People like getting "likes" on Facebook and like comments even better. It may also show who your real friends are.

Sometimes I don't feel like I'm making progress, so sometimes I'll vent on my own page or the special page I created. Someone usually responds back with an encouraging comment ("You're doing great, keep going for it!") and just one nice comment is something that will help you through another day.

Mark's Basic Idea Number Three: Set a goal AND a reward for losing weight.

As part of the goal, set up a big REWARD or BET that if you complete the goal, you will buy something nice, or do something that you've always wanted to do, or something else.

Now, at the time of this writing, I have not hit my goal yet, 100 pounds. But I've got a little encouragement. In our household, we're very cautious on our spending and our budget. We drive plain, utilitarian cars. My wife and I dream of getting a "fun" car, but she'd kill me if I went out and bought one at the drop of a hat.

However, I discussed my goal with my wife, and agreed that if I can lose 100 pounds and keep it off for a month, I can go get whatever car I want (within a certain price range). So I want something like this:

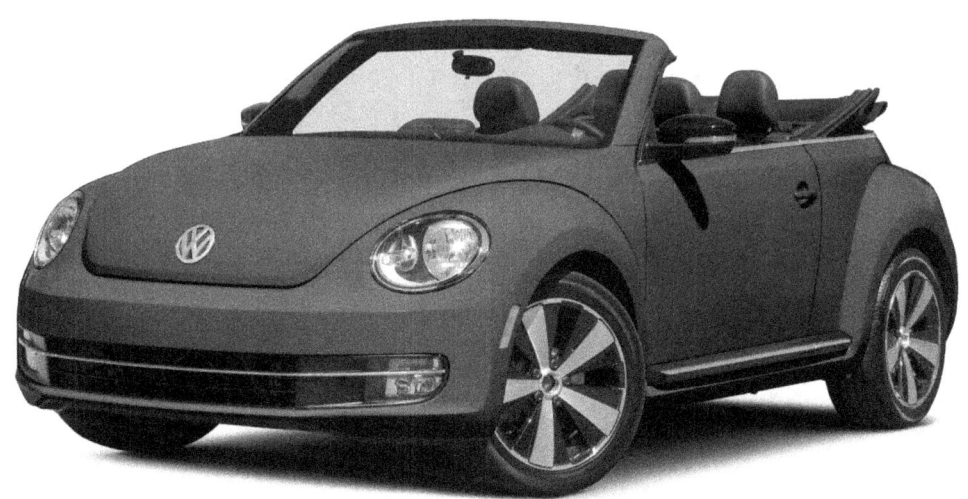

Yup, a fun VW Beetle (Picture courtesy of newscars.com).

(Special note, as of the date of this writing, VW is having a scandal with their diesel cars, so I might rethink this car...)

So it's a little bit like waiting for Christmas, or a birthday, or something big where there's a prize at the end. Otherwise, doing this weight loss doesn't do anything for me, even with an ego boost, better health, and lots of compliments.

Maybe you can promise yourself a vacation if you accomplish your weight goal. Maybe buy a boat. Or a motorcycle. SOMETHING.

I post pictures of this Beetle and other Beetles in my office cubicle, I use Beetles as screensaver images on my computer, and so on, I just constantly remind myself what I WILL get WHEN I achieve this goal.

Mark's Basic Idea Number Four: Track what you eat, when, and how much, and track what you weigh.

This is going to be variable, considering there are several different programs, facilities, classes, groups and other weight control programs. Many of this will implement some sort of tracking like this. The company that I use has their own journal (filled with blank forms) that you put in what you weigh, what your blood pressure is (taken by the staff), and you fill in what you ate, how much (servings or ounces or grams, or whatever). It also enables you to track and follow what you're doing right or wrong, or if you had much or too little of a certain food. As for tracking WEIGHT, that's another matter. Only track and log what you weigh in at when you meet with your group or clinic or class, at least a once or twice a week. We'll be talking about this a little more later in the book.

Sometimes the tracking will help you compare some days to others when you are looking at trends, behaviors, and eating patterns. For example, I'll notice that my weight loss will slow down if I'm eating later at night. You can try experimenting for a week to see if you eat earlier it changes, and test eating later to see what works and what doesn't.

The journals/logbooks used can also track physical activity if you're so inclined.

Some of the science, good, bad, and otherwise

Now as I mentioned at the beginning, a lot of what I learned and am going to put out there now is a combination of personal experience and bits and pieces of actual science and/or other authorities.

What I really DON'T want to do is take 50 pages to explain how a piece of buzzard meat gets metabolized in your digestive system. I've had enough of those books. I also had enough of 30 minute videos that tells me what could have been said in only 3 minutes.

I'll have a list of sources at the end of the book, basically not by the exact specific page, but rather some articles and some books that you can read entirely at your leisure if you want to do that. Again, this is what I DID, not necessarily what everyone SHOULD do. It worked for me, your mileage may vary, yadda yadda yadda….

The resource section at the end of this book will cover a lot of the in-depth information. Now I'll admit this is being lazy, but I do this for a point. That is, some people want to learn about how everything works in it's entirety and then find out what the ultimate single thing you have to take from that information. Here, I bring you the "single points" and if you're really that curious, investigate the research, info, and theory behind it all at your own pace.

Mark's Basic Idea Number Five: Eat too much or without limits and you'll gain weight.

Well, DUH, right? But I'm serious, and that is, the weight programs that are available, the one I'm on (an unnamed company), Weight Watchers, Jenny Craig, and several others set limits as to what you can/should eat. That is, eat only X amount of certain foods each day.

On the program that I'm on, I was set for a limit of 3 vegetables, 3 fruits, 3 proteins, 1 fat, 2 dairy, and 2 "starches". (Later I would be adjusted to 4 vegetables, 3 fruits, 2 proteins, 1 fat, 1 dairy, and 2 starches.)

Basically what I'm saying is that you can NOT ever go back to just grabbing a large bag of potato chips or Doritos or whatever and sit and mindlessly eat. Same goes for opening a full pint of Haagen Dazs and just sitting there gobbling spoonful after spoonful (you DO know the recommended amount of servings for one of those containers is THREE AND A HALF servings, right?). That is, the proper amount is probably just the first ¾ of an inch from the top when you open it.

This was something I had to make a humongous effort to get used to. Other members of my family still eat like this. What do to?

Plain and simple, you're probably eating to avoid some boredom, like watching TV. What worked for me was simply getting either a glass of water or something relatively safe to eat and only a controlled amount of it, like a piece of string cheese, or a very limited amount of air-popped popcorn. Or have sex. Can't eat and have sex unless you...er, well....

In other words, you can lose a lot simply with portion control. Only eat out measured portions. Or, do what I do, I cook individual servings of food for myself and put them in single containers in the fridge.

Now if you have a family meal all together, that's a little hard, if there's a whole plate of multiple pieces of fried chicken, where you can pick one piece, five, or all 12 or whatever. You just have to limit yourself.

Now again, the program that I'm on and several other programs (WW, JC) will offer what your servings should be and what amounts/weights they should be. A proper serving of any form of beef should be about 4 ounces (yes, a quarter pound). Chicken, about six ounces, and fish about 8, but these are rough estimates and they will vary on the type of meat. But I'll get into meat in a little while. It's just an example that you have to get in your head as to what a "single serving" really means and having to stick with it. Yes, a quarter pound burger patty DOES count, but you can't have the bun...or the cheese...or ketchup...(more on protein later).

Mark's Basic Idea Number Six: Almost anything sweet is NOT your friend.

First, we tackle the obvious: Anything with sugar added or has sugar as an ingredient is going to be bad. Aside from tooth decay, as most of us learned as a kid, sugar, through our digestive system DOES go to your fat cells.

According to the National Council on Strength and Fitness, the two most common sources of carbohydrates most of us in this country eat are high-fructose corn syrup and sucrose. These refined sugars, which are added to many foods, lack the vitamins, minerals, proteins and fiber found in complex carbohydrates. These "empty calories" can cause blood sugar levels to spike, which in turn causes insulin levels to rise. Insulin is a hormone released by the body that helps regulate blood sugar levels. If sugar is not quickly used for energy, insulin removes it from the blood, and it is then converted into triglycerides in the liver. These triglycerides can then be stored as body fat.

In other words, sugar will cause fat. No two butts about it.

What about fruit, doesn't that contain sugar or sugars as well? It's a different sugar,

Simply put, they all contain sugars, but with different amounts and types. The main two are fructose and sucrose, but each different fruit has differing amounts. Again, the process of handling sugars in fruit is very similar to straight table sugar, but that's an oversimplification. Low sugar fruits include strawberries, pineapple, cantaloupe, melons, most anything with the "berry" name in it. Apples are the middle ground, having plenty (almost too much) sugar, but having enough fiber to be of an offset to the sugar. But higher sugar fruits include bananas, grapes, mangoes, and pomegranates.

You get essential nutrients, vitamins, and all that from fruits, however, just try to keep the fruits low in sugar as you can.

So that's obvious. Now about the NOT so obvious. What about sugar-free foods? What about diet soda? Those can be bad as well.

Studies are showing that people that consume a lot of "sugar free" products cause people to gain weight as well. Some thought that the problem was that people were mentally justifying eating or drinking other things in excess because they're supposedly not eating any sugar, right? Maybe...

Two BIG problems are being discovered nowadays in regards to what sugar substitutes and artificial sweeteners do to the body:

1) Some studies suggest that the brain, upon tasting and consuming something sweet, will tell the body to react as though it's receiving actual sugar. The brain tells the body it thinks it's getting sugar and it acts accordingly. Blood sugar levels spike even after people consume some of the more common substitutes like aspartame and sucralose.

2) A more recent set of studies also show that gut bacteria is changed after having consumed a lot of artificial sweeteners. Gut bacteria is basically the active things in your guts that help process and digest food, but it can go out of balance. At first it was noticed that the gut bacteria was higher and different in people that consumed artificial sweeteners and were overweight. But after giving them a specific type of antibiotic, the gut bacteria then came down to levels of those like normal people.

In other words, the studies are starting to come through that show artificial sweeteners don't really help. More testing and comparisons are going on with other sweeteners that have been on the market, such as Stevia, to see if they spike blood sugar and cause other weight-gaining effects. Results look good, however, the jury is still out.

But rather than take a risk, don't try to consume any of them anyway. Be SURE to read product labels on foods.

Mark's Basic Idea Number Seven: Carbs are not your friend.

When Dr Atkin's "low carb" diet became popular, the basic science proved that eating carbohydrates and sugar led to fat, not eating fat leading to fat. It also did away with the calorie counting or the "calories in/calories out" theory of diet and nutrition. This is actually catching up with more mainstream diet plan providers, as the science behind it is also being more generally accepted.

Carbs and sugars basically get consumed and if they're not used immediately (like if you're going to run a mile or do anything physical), they get added to body fat. But proteins and fats actually cause the body to "work" at digesting, and doesn't go directly to fat. Fats in foods help deliver nutrients and vitamins to the body and brain, so you need to eat SOME fats. Protein builds muscle and does other good things. Now most fruits and vegetables have carbohydrates in them, but again, some deliver that in the form of digesting to sugars. We will get to veggies shortly.

I'll say this much, in MY own personal experience, I had lost about 45 pounds on a low-carb diet, but I had other issues at the time and didn't continue onward, but that basically works as well.

The basic carbs to avoid are:

- All breads
- Potatoes
- Rice
- Corn
- Peas
- Pasta
- Anything from wheat in general
- Anything made from rice or corn in general

Now what exactly is counted as "low carb", or what is too many? In the original *Dr Atkin's Diet Revolution*, total carbs of a given food per serving is basically:

Total carbs in grams - fiber (in grams) - sugar alcohols (in grams) = Net carbs

There is some disagreement between the Atkins corporation and other sources of nutrition (WedMD, and others) indicating you can probably only subtract HALF the sugar alcohols because some of them, not all, still act like real sugars.

The Atkins program, when it was first released, suggested that you try to keep your total carbs in a day under 50 grams.

Here's a simple example:

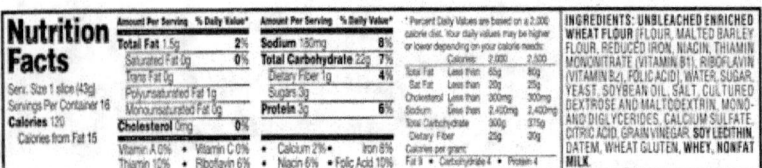

(Courtesy Fooducate.com)

In one slice, we have:

Total carbs, 22g - Fiber, 1g = 21g Net carbs.

But this is just ONE slice, if you want a sandwich, you gotta have two slices and that will put you at 42 grams already and that's just one sandwich in one meal.

Again, if you can keep away from a LOT of the carbs, you'll do fine.

Mark's Basic Idea Number Eight: Most vegetables are okay, the more the better.

That being said, you saw in the previous section that a FEW vegetables are bad, mostly the starchy, carb-laden ones. All vegetables have some carbs and fiber, but mostly you need to stay away from potatoes, corn, and peas.

Fresh is better, frozen is okay, but canned is not preferable. This is mostly because of the processing, salts, and possibly oils added to canned veggies that can be harmful. No, I won't get into the discussion of chemical can liners (Bisphenol A, BPA), the concern here is mostly the salts and preservatives that they may add.

If you are a big veggie fan, then you can almost eat any of them to your heart's content. But you may have to watch how you COOK them. Boiling is ok, or a stir-fry using as little oil as possible, or using a non-stick spray (PAM) will work. Just don't go overboard on the oil. No, you can't bread them and/or deep-fry them, the calories and fats will to off the chart.

Green vegetables are preferred, spinach, broccoli, kale, lettuce, etc, but the more dark green they are the better as they have more nutrients.

A few veggies are in-between having no sugar and having too much, carrots can actually produce too much sugars if you really eat more than usual in one sitting. But in general, they're less blood-sugar-spiking than say a couple baked potatoes.

If you figure that eating salads may be the best way to go, try to go for spinach and kale salads, as most type of lettuce (iceberg, romaine) are less nutritious. But take it easy on the salad dressing, typically no more than 2 ounces of any standard dressing (regular or lo-fat). If you can enjoy a salad with an olive oil, again, that's okay, but don't drown your salad in it.

But I don't go into a lot of detail here because I'm not really a vegetable fan. I've mostly had carrots and celery to eat through the day (taking them to work for my lunch and supper). But I have a spinach/kale salad every day, making this a bit more helpful and tasty, but I add whatever meat/protein (see next section) to the salad to make it more interesting.

Mark's Basic Idea Number Nine: Fat doesn't necessarily go directly into your own fat, but go ahead and load up on protein

Try to cut down fats, but it's not as bad as carbs.

You need SOME fats to process nutrients, it's good for the brain as well. But briefly, too much fat can cause problems and not get consumed.

But there's the whole counter-intuitive issue of "are low fat foods all that helpful"? That is, in order to reduce the fats in foods, the producers of such food have to add chemicals or sugars or other things that are still not good for your body to process. That's usually the problem with mostly processed foods.

But if you can get lean meats, like ground beef that's over 90% lean versus cheap hamburger at 80% lean, that will help. Turkey and chicken, even better, and most fish are better yet. Tuna in a CAN is okay, but only if packed in water and if it has minimal amounts of bad things (salt, sugars, check the label!).

A low-fat ice-cream may be a good example of where they may take out the fat, but add sugars and other things to make it taste "almost as good" as the real stuff.

The interaction with most fats in your foods is in your blood stream, but the real damage with fats is that they can clog your arteries and raise your cholesterol and cause problems with your heart or other organs.

Get lower fat foods and check out their food labels compared to standard foods and stick to leaner meats if possible. The program that I'm on roughly states specific limits for fats and specific amount of meats to eat. 8 ounces of milk per day (skim preferred) is what I'm mostly under, low fat mozzarella cheese is allowed, but only one string cheese stick per day. On the meats, usually around 4 to 5 ounces for beef, pork, 5-6 for chicken and turkey, and up to about 8 for most fish, per serving, again, I currently eat about 2 servings of meats.

On a related note, on proteins, the body takes more effort to consume proteins that it does for fats and sugars. In fact the body expends more calories in comparison in just digesting meat. Amounts vary as suggested in the previous paragraph. There are several table and charts on the web that you can use to pick out the best bang for the buck, but in general you can try to get roughly 30 grams of protein in a serving or more and that will help.

Some people, or even more, celebrities, have gone to swigging protein shakes and powders with the thought being that as you consume more protein, your body will work that much harder to digest. Actually in the amounts that people will try to overuse protein powders, it will build more muscle and actually make you heavier. It would definitely help if you were going for more muscle definition or building more of a bodybuilder's physique. But on almost EVERY protein powder is the instruction "DO NOT USE FOR LOSING WEIGHT". Some powders will have sweeteners (as mentioned before) that are in direct conflict with you trying to stay away from them.

Mark's Basic Idea Number Ten: Stay off salt/sodium

Stay off added salt, stay off any heavily salted foods. No bacon, no bacon bits, no ham, no beef jerky, and for that matter, most fast foods will do you in.

The main emphasis on salt in regards to a weight-loss diet is that you can retain water and of course make you heavier.   However, too much salt causes problems with blood pressure and kidney function. Better to stay off salt if possible.

Well, of course that's rather depressing, many foods are rather bland without salt and are no fun to eat. So we start looking at salt alternatives, such as the commercially popular Mrs. Dash, and several other brands of alternative salt.

Mrs Dash and others like it throw OTHER kinds of spices and ingredients that make your food have SOME sort of taste. Some other substitutes use Potassium, but the drawbacks to Potassium-based substitutes are (1) the metallic taste and (2) conflicts with some blood pressure medications. But the potassium ones may work for you, your mileage may vary.

If you're checking labels, the maximum amount of sodium a person should have is about 1500 milligrams in one day. But looking at food labels can be downright scary. A beef jerky stick can have upwards of 1000 by itself. One 3 ounce piece of ham can have 900 mg. One HALF of a teaspoon of soy sauce can have 1300 milligrams!

In my own experience, I was following my program and it did specifically state to try and not use salt, but I didn't pay attention to it at first. After running into some plateaus, I had sat down with my clinic's staff and we tried looking for things that I might not be doing right. Sure enough, I wasn't paying attention to my salt consumption. After cutting off salt right away, I had a quick drop and that helped break my plateau. But of course that was just me, and perhaps there still might have been other factors involved.

Mark's Basic Idea Number Eleven: Exercise is good for you of course, but it's not the total solution

Basically, some experts suggest that 80% of a weight control program is food consumption and 20% is exercise. Well, I'll be honest, I'm mostly doing only the food consumption.

Now, as of this writing, I've lost about 75 pounds so far with just food portion control. The program that I'm on does not emphasize exercise. If you DO exercise, great. Knock yourself out. But don't be overly concerned. Getting any more physical activity is a plus. Some programs may suggest that you do "X" amount of physical activity per day or every other day. That's great.

I'll admit it. I'd rather sit on a rabid porcupine than to do any exercise. I've several bad experiences as a child in regards to physical activity, P.E. classes in school, and generally not being comfortable or not tolerating physical discomfort in exercising. Hate it.

However what I HAVE discovered is that after losing a bit of weight, I've been able to do more physically around the house and out about town. Taking long walks don't bother me as much as when I used to weigh over 300 pounds. Setting up and tearing down band equipment as a musician also is easier now and I can more more stuff quickly than ever, so I am getting a little more activity.

But, from the reading and research that I've done, the science at least does prove that if you exercise more, your metabolism increases and you consume the foods you eat faster and you burn more fat. Just carrying more muscle burns more calories than carrying fat. It's something like 13 calories get burned for each pound of muscle you are carrying, versus about 3 for each pound of fat. But it's also known that exercising can make you hungrier, hence the temptation to eat or OVEReat can come and defeat the purpose of you exercising to begin with. Just be careful.

As for the HOW to get you started and continuing on an exercise program, I cannot suggest a lot of things except try to find ANY kind of exercise that, I would say, is the least objectionable. You may not like running, how about long walks instead? You might not aerobic exercise, but anaerobic exercise, such as weightlifting, may appeal to you more. You can join a gym, but also check out your local recreation center in your city or town. Maybe weekly volleyball? Badminton? Walleyball? Swimming? Whatever. I did some walking around a lap track at my local recreation center and that suited me just fine. (I ought to get back to that....)

Mark's Basic Idea Number Twelve: To maintain your sanity, one "cheat meal" a week can help make the long-running process of weight loss easier to continue

Some programs, including the one I attend, <u>really don't suggest doing this.</u> The basic problem here is that one "cheat meal" might lead to a "cheat day" and even worse, lead to a "cheat month" and before you know it, you've given up on the diet.

Let's go back to putting this in a plan. That is, PLAN your cheat meal and allow yourself to have one small cheat. No, that does NOT mean you get to replace your Friday night proper meal with plowing down a whole bag of Doritos, or a whole pint of Haagen-Dazs. No, you can probably pick something simple, but not in over-excess like a slice of pizza, or maybe a baked potato, or just a regular sandwich with real bread. Nothing big. It's a little bit of consolation if trying to follow all of the above ideas get to be a little much and you need a break.

Actually I try to take it one step further and get a "cheat" meal only if I happen to set a new low weight for the week. If I make it, I get a small reward. If not, I try harder and look forward to the goal and the small reward.

Speaking of weights:

Mark's Basic Idea Number Thirteen: Get a good scale, but only weigh yourself every few days or every WEEK, don't weigh yourself every day

Weighing yourself every day has one basic problem: You'll obsess over what you might have done WRONG over the last 24 hours on your diet and get yourself depressed because of it. This is a long run, not a sprint. You do best by weighing yourself periodically, but over a longer amount of time so you get a good average loss and can see progress easier.

In weighing yourself every day and if you notice a weight INCREASE on a particular day, you'll worry and say to yourself, "Did that 2 pieces of toast cause my 3 pound upswing?", or, "Maybe I should not have had that extra piece of fish!", or, "I HAD A COOKIE AND I GAINED 5 POUNDS!!! ARGH!!!!".

You'll get overly concerned over things that may or may NOT have an effect on your weight. Your body is constantly operating and processing foods, your blood flow, your heart rate, and your digestive systems are all doing things simultaneously, but over a longer time to affect everything with your weight. General knowledge suggests that anything you eat will take 2 to 4 days to process through your whole digestive system. So what you eat or don't eat will take a few days anyway, so a day-by-day weigh in won't be able to tell you much in terms of progress.

The program that I'm on has you weigh in at least 3 times a week, basically assuming that you might space out your weigh-in's at once nearly every two days. That's about as close together as I would allow for it.

What to do now that you're there?

That is, if you've accomplished your goal of losing X number of pounds, how do you stay at your weight and keep off the weight? Indeed several studies and experiments have been done that say that most folks do gain some of or all their weight back.

As of now, I don't have the ultimate answer, except that for the plan and the clinic that I'm using is offering to me, I still stay to a specific plan and "add" foods and portions and try to keep the weight stabilized.

It's mostly going to be a matter of staying on a healthy pattern of eating and/or exercising from now on until I DIE. That may be hard. What I'm hoping for myself is that I'll just stay on an eating pattern and try to keep on it as though I'm actively in weight-loss mode.

One of the major things that led to me being heavy was the habit I had of sitting and mindlessly eating out of a whole bag of potato chips and the pint of Haagen-Dazs. I know I can't do that anymore so I've got to establish that as a good habit. If I still feel like I want to eat or have anything in my mouth, I'll usually now go for a glass of water with ice.

Some programs (clinics, WW, JC) may have extended programs, or "maintenance" programs in which if you feel that you're drifting up in weight, you can go back and they can help get you back on track.

Epilogue:

Well there you have it.

Now, as for the experiences, I'll get into a few things when I started.

I bought a food scale, it measures ounces and grams, and my plan that I followed mostly had serving sizes measured in ounces, so that worked out fine.

During the few couple months, simply limiting portion size and amounts did most of the weight loss. I also stopped doing any "unlimited" eating, like picking up a bag of Doritos and mindlessly eating until whenever.

How did I do? This might help:

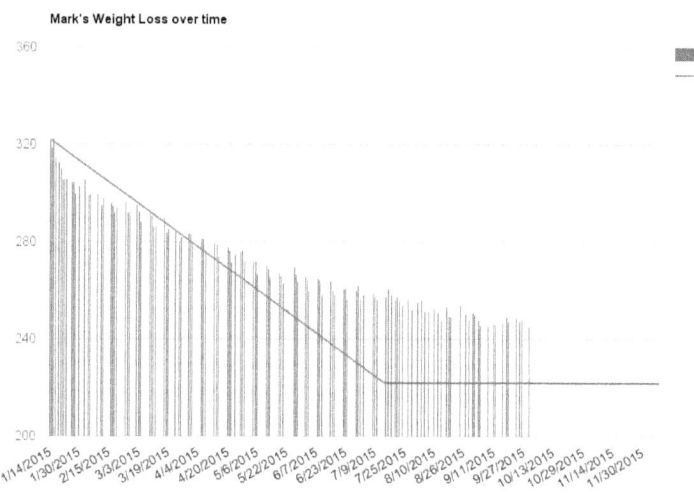

Mark's Weight Loss over time

Notice the big drop at first over the first few months as again, it was mostly portion control that was the cause. But it slowed down a bit and I'd fret over foods, what I ate, and what happened after I DID eat. Then my body would indeed start getting picky and it seemed like if I did eat the wrong thing at one time, I'd either plateau or gain a little. That didn't happen much, but the plateauing would occur more often now than earlier.

I would usually weigh in on Monday and Tuesday evenings, then on Wednesday mornings. If I managed to reach a new "low" weight, I would then have my cheat meal right after that, such that it would be consumed and digested right away before I went to work (I would work Wednesday afternoons and evenings).

The program that I'm on emphasizes eating, drinking, or consuming at least something every 2-½ to 3 hours. This is not quite scientifically proven, just Google "eating frequent small meals diet". The idea is that your metabolism, if kept constantly active, will also continue to run at a certain pace and continue to burn your fat as well. Sounds good, and some folks will proclaim this is true for them. But science hasn't really proved that out. At least the real reason it MIGHT work is that you have small meals that added together over the course of a day, you might consume less in total. Or at least if you do eat often and in small portions, you won't all of a sudden eat a TON at the next meal because you feel starved. This also lends credence to the long-time theory that it's just "total calories" that matter.

The other thing that along with this is that the experts at my clinic don't want you to starve yourself, claiming that your metabolism will stop as well. You might be able to fast (not eat for a longer time) for like a day, and it might give you a quick drop, but it's not a long-term strategy from what I've been doing. There is also a danger that fasting can burn off muscle instead of fat, including heart tissue. Not a good thing.

How did I deal with temptations and urges to go off the wagon? It was pretty much a combination of (1) keeping my eye on the price, as earlier, remembering what I will promise I'll treat myself when I lose all the weight, (2) planning the cheat meal and remembering that, (3) usually reaching for a glass of water, and (4) admittedly, sheer will power. I know, #4 isn't going to be the ultimate prevention, but the other three help more.

From the multiple programs that are out there, one is a "5 days eating and 2 day fasting" diet known as the "5:2 Diet", and it's found here: http://thefastdiet.co.uk/. Basically you eat fairly normally for 5 days, and fast for 2 days (consecutively or non-consecutively). On the fasting days you eat about 500 calories instead of the normal 2000 to 2400 calories that most women and men are suggested to eat, respectively. If you were to try this, I'd strongly suggest most of the points I made above, that is, do it with an organized group that can cheer you on and help you track what works. I've attempted this one, but didn't follow it faithfully on my own.

Back to the clinic program that I'm on, it's mostly set up as "this is the most stuff you can eat for this category" and still continue to lose weight. This program is really marketed (in my opinion) to casual suburban housewives or pre-retirees that have a lot less metabolism and don't want to give up anything in terms of all their favorite foods like bread and sweet snacks. The program that I'm on actually wants you to eat "2 starches" a day, which is basically a single light english muffin or two pieces of light (less than 40 calories bread). I would ask the program staff, if bread is not that good for you, why not just NOT eat it? They claim that you still need a little of each food group to keep what they think is a balanced diet.

To me, it's like you can be a lot healthier by quitting smoking entirely, not just change from regular cigarettes to low-tar, light cigarettes. Don't eat just a little bread, just cut out the bread, or rice, or potatoes entirely.

To be more cynical, the program I use also SELLS (and I capitalize that as well) products like "healthy" protein shake powders and snack bars and they're pretty damn expensive. Again, this is along the theory that at least if you portion-control everything, including the bad stuff, you'll still lose weight. I've looked at the ingredients and nutrition labels for the powders and bars and they contain sugars, sugar alcohols, and artificial sweeteners. The only thing that I've really found the powders good for is for making smoothies with vegetables to make the smoothies sweet and tolerable.

Smoothies? It's a step in the right direction and if it helps you consume more vegetables, the better, but again, we get into adding any kind of sweetener might do more damage than you need. That, and some veggies don't blend all that well. I've tried kale and lettuce, run through a Ninja blender to make a smoothie, but the problems are (1) the pulverized veggies are still gritty and (2) the taste of the vegetable can still overpower whatever you put in to make it sweet (if any). Fruit smoothies are good too, but I was combining them with the powders. I've had mixed results, mostly that I'd plateau or stall if I consumed smoothies the day before a weigh-in.

So what i mostly do for smoothies now is simply just use straight fruit, ice, and water, and I run them through a Ninja (brand) blender. I use no powders or sweeteners. If you balance out the ice just right, you can make them slightly thicker than a margarita and enjoy them more. Strawberry smoothies are just about right.

Speaking of drinks, my program really pushes "no alcohol", they're just "liquid calories" (or "liquid carbs") and any form of consuming alcohol is bad. I mostly consume beer in infrequent times and amounts. (Mostly when I play music at bars and events, but not much more than that....okay, maybe at band practice...)

The program really tried to emphasize that I stick with their list of X proteins, Y veggies, Z fruits, Q starches, and P fats, and 2 dairy (or 1 now) and that they can't guarantee their weight loss results unless I follow their program to the letter. So it's been a bit hard doing what they want, and really trying to follow the more correct and successful science behind real weight loss. But I've tried a few things that were out of bounds for a few days, such as skipping or fasting.

I've also found that consuming everything earlier seems to help because you will actively consume and digest it if you're up and around at work or doing things at home during the day. If you consume a big meal late in the day (dinner, supper, or whatever you call it), the food will just sit and not digest enough for the next morning if I go in for a weigh in.

Speaking of weigh-ins, I will usually fast or not eat anything in the morning if I arrive at my clinic at their opening time. Then I get weighed and THEN have breakfast. That will at least show my lowest weight for the day. Not what my clinic prefers, but at least it's a good time to aim for an "all time low" and it helps a little bit mentally.

There's the theory that drinking at least 8 eight-ounce glasses of water will also help lose weight. Or drinking 8 12-ounce glasses. Or just drinking "lots" of water, period. There are not a lot of supporting evidence that it leads to weight loss, but at least drinking a lot of water is healthy in general.

One supposed reason, with only a few studies, is that the body expends some energy (calories) in consuming cold water. I've really not noticed any difference in drinking a lot of water versus what I think is a "normal" amount of water.

That all said about drinking water, I clearly drink too much Diet Coke and that's actually a bigger challenge than losing weight. Considering the section previously about sweet foods and drinks, this is still an obstacle I'm trying to get over. I've noticed a "little" difference between days that I drink about 4 of them in a day and going cold turkey the other days. I do lose a little more on the days before I weigh in, but it's still hard. Supposedly Tipper Gore (former wife of Al), lost weight after Al's 2000 presidential campaign by "simply stopped drinking diet soda". Your mileage may vary. I still work at this.

Other sources suggest that if you eat only non-processed food, regardless of the food type, you will be healthier. Basically, no prepared meats like breakfast sausage, bacon, pre-cooked patties, even processed veggie patties. This is mostly because chemicals are supposedly evil and many will have excessive salt and fat. True, you can avoid some sugars, artificial sweeteners, salt, and processed fats. This is a lot of how most of my food is in the current plan that I use, I cook my own meats, mostly and get fresh vegetables and fruits (frozen can be okay if you check the labels to watch for anything added).

Along those lines is Jonathan Bailor and the SANE diet. It's mostly a program in that it simply directs you to eat mostly vegetables, a portion of protein (meat, fish, etc), a little bit of fruit, and that's about it. But he also goes the route of pushing protein powder, but using those that have low sugars/sweeteners, but under this program (about 50 grams of protein per serving), the informal attempts that I've tried to use to see if this works, didn't work for me, and in fact, as I mentioned in the section about protein, most powders are specifically labelled "do not use for weight loss".

In summary: A lot of this entire book is just a collection of things that I learned and/or found that work, or DON'T WORK in reducing weight.

I really want to make the first couple of points very important: You may be a strong person, mentally and physically, but getting assistance and enlisting support in your weight loss is VITAL. Some people can do it alone, but in my own experience, having support and having guidance in doing this works for me. I hope it can work for you.

My weight loss has been a little on the slow side, compared to how the program that I was originally on gave me some overly optimistic estimates. They HAVE had different clients that have lost 100 pounds in half a year, but that almost comes down to 4 pounds a week, which some doctors I've spoken with suggest that may be too fast. For me it's closer to 1.5 to 2 pounds a week. Your results may vary and even then, you're probably eating stuff that's better for you overall anyway.

If at least I gave you something new to think about doing differently in losing weight, then I've done my job. At the end of most diet books I've felt a little encouraged, some of them not so much. At least here, I'm not trying to push a specific diet "plan" or "fad" on you. With Atkins, the Paleo diets, SANE, or just about anything else out there, they share a few common themes in terms of food content. What I hope that some of you DO get is that at least you get some support, find programs that help you be accountable for your weight loss activity, and stay away from the obvious bad stuff or bad habits.

This books DEFINITELY will be revised repeatedly as I expect to hear back from friends, relatives, doctors, and complete strangers about any information that I've put out there that's just not quite right, or oversimplified, or just flat-out WRONG.

I actively encourage you to contact me for right now through my Facebook page: https://www.facebook.com/MarkLoses100lbs

Good luck!

References, resources, and places where I found stuff about diets and dieting:

SANE Solution diet: http://sanesolution.com/

Atkins diet: http://www.atkins.com/

WedMD, where I got most of my specific info on fruits, vegetables, water consumption: http:/www.webmd.com

Mayo Clinic, another good source of science-based info on nutrition and diets: http://www.mayoclinic.org/

Bliss Returned, a blog that happens to have a good reference list of sugars in fruits and vegetables: https://blissreturned.wordpress.com/2012/02/05/fruits-and-vegetable-list-of-low-and-high-sugar-fruit-and-vegetable/

The Paleo Diet, but this link has more fruits and vegetable information: http://thepaleodiet.com/fruits-and-sugars/

Weight Watchers: http://www.weightwatchers.com

Jenny Craig: http://www.jennycraig.com

The TIME article that offers information about diet soda and weight gain: http://time.com/3746047/diet-soda-bad-belly-fat/

More food label info: www.fooducate.com